Hypnotherapy

A Beginner's Guide to Practicing Hypnotherapy, Methods and Techniques

Dani Twain

Copyright Notice

All rights reserved. No part of this publication may be reproduced, stored in a retrieval system or transmitted in any form or by any means, including electronic, digital, mechanical, photocopying, audio recording, printing or otherwise, without written permission from the publisher or the author.

Contents

COPYRIGHT

CHAPTER 1

Understanding Hypnosis

Hypnosis and Sleep: What's the Difference?

The History of Hypnosis

Myths About Hypnosis

Types of Hypnosis

When is Hypnosis Used?

Who Should Not Use Hypnosis?

How Does a Hypnotherapy Session Work?

Pros and Cons of Hypnosis

How to Tell If Someone Is Hypnotized

CHAPTER 2

The Power of Self-Hypnosis

The Impact of Self-Hypnosis

How Self-Hypnosis Works

Self-Hypnosis in Medical Treatments

How to Hypnotize

CHAPTER 3

Understanding Hypnotherapy

What is Hypnotherapy?

The Difference Between Classical and Ericksonian Hypnosis

How a Hypnotherapy Session Works

CHAPTER 4

Hypnotic Trance

Exploring Dissociation, Absorption, and Suggestibility

Exploring Different Depths of Hypnosis

Chapter 1

Understanding Hypnosis

Many people have doubts about hypnosis, much like they do about mind-reading or magic tricks, like sawing a girl in half on stage. However, hypnosis can help people quickly and effectively overcome bad habits, addictions, and negative thoughts without needing strong medications or other heavy treatments.

Let's dive into what hypnosis is, who created it, what problems it can solve, and who should avoid it.

What is Hypnosis?

Hypnosis is a state where you feel very relaxed and highly focused at the same time. During hypnosis, your critical thinking, the part of your mind that evaluates and judges things, takes a break. This makes you more open to suggestions, new ideas, and changes in behavior or habits.

Here are some key features of a hypnotic state:

- Altered State of Consciousness: Your attention is intensely focused on one thing, such as the voice of a hypnotherapist, while your awareness of everything else around you becomes less clear.

- **Increased Suggestibility:** You become more open to accepting new ideas or suggestions.

- **Changed Perception of Time:** Time may seem to move slower or faster than usual.

We often experience a state similar to hypnosis, called an "everyday trance," several times a day (anywhere from 5 to 30 times, according to studies). For instance, when you're deeply absorbed in a book, you may not notice what's happening around you. Or when you're on a bus, lost in thought while watching the scenery go by, you might miss your stop. These moments are like mini-hypnosis sessions where we become deeply focused and detached from our surroundings.

Hypnosis and Sleep: What's the Difference?

At one point, people thought hypnosis was a form of sleep. The word "hypnosis" even comes from the Greek word for sleep, "hypnos." Ivan Pavlov, a famous Russian scientist, believed that when a person listened to repetitive sounds, like a hypnotist's voice, a part of their brain would become inactive. This calmness would then spread across the brain, with only one area staying active to communicate with the hypnotist.

But as science progressed, it became clear that hypnosis and sleep are not the same at all.

In a state of hypnosis, a person is aware of their surroundings and can respond to the hypnotist's suggestions. The brain is very active, especially in areas responsible for decision-making and focus. Physically, the person is relaxed, but their mind stays alert. On the other hand, during sleep, a person is unconscious and unaware of their surroundings. The brain goes through different stages of activity, and muscle tone decreases, making the person unaware of their physical state.

Hypnosis is a technique used to achieve specific goals, such as therapy or overcoming bad habits. Sleep, however, is a natural process that we need to rest and recover.

The History of Hypnosis

People have known about hypnosis since ancient times. In places like Egypt, Greece, and Rome, hypnosis-like states were used in religious rituals. Similar practices were found among people in Siberia, Tibet, and South America. However, these practices were forgotten over time until the 18th century when hypnosis made a comeback.

Key Moments in Hypnosis History

In the late 18th century, an Austrian doctor named Franz Anton Mesmer developed a theory called "animal magnetism" or mesmerism. He believed that a magnetic force flowed through the human body and could be controlled to induce a trance-like state. Mesmer's ideas were further developed by his student, Armand-Marie-Jacques de Chastenet, Marquis de Puysegur, who called the trance state "artificial somnambulism."

In 1842, a Scottish surgeon named James Braid coined the term "hypnosis," derived from the Greek word for sleep. He initially thought hypnosis was related to a state of focused attention and relaxation similar to sleep.

In the late 19th century, a French neurologist named Jean-Martin Charcot used hypnosis to study and treat neurological disorders, especially hysteria. His work helped establish hypnosis as a psychological tool. Charcot's student, Pierre Janet, focused on the psychological aspects of hypnosis and its potential for therapy.

Ambroise Auguste Liébeault, a French physician, is considered the father of modern hypnotherapy. He developed techniques to promote mental healing without drugs, founding a hypnosis school in Nancy. Liébeault emphasized the importance of a positive therapeutic environment filled with trust and acceptance for successful treatment.

By the late 19th and early 20th centuries, hypnosis had gained recognition as a legitimate medical practice and was incorporated into mainstream psychology and psychiatry.

Myths About Hypnosis

Like many things that are mysterious and hard to understand, hypnosis has sparked a lot of myths. Let's clear up some of these misconceptions.

Myth: Hypnosis is mind control.

Reality: Hypnosis is not mind control. It's a state where a person is very focused and open to suggestions. However, the person can choose to accept or reject these suggestions.

Myth: Only weak-minded or gullible people can be hypnotized.

Reality: Hypnosis is a natural state that anyone can experience, regardless of intelligence or personality. Being able to be hypnotized doesn't mean a person is weak or gullible; it varies from person to person.

Myth: You can suggest anything to a person in a state of hypnosis.

Reality: In a hypnotic state, people are still in control and will not accept suggestions that go against their beliefs or values. They can reject anything that feels wrong to them.

Myth: Hypnosis is a form of sleep or unconsciousness.

Reality: While people under hypnosis might seem relaxed and less aware of their surroundings, they are actually awake and able to respond to suggestions from the hypnotist.

Myth: Hypnosis is used only for entertainment.

Reality: Hypnosis is not just for stage shows. It's also a valuable tool for therapy, helping people with issues like anxiety, phobias, weight loss, and quitting smoking.

Types of Hypnosis

Hypnosis comes in various forms, each with its own methods and uses. Here are some common types:

Classic Hypnosis

Classic or traditional hypnosis is directive and authoritarian. The hypnotherapist takes the lead, giving clear instructions and guiding the client through commands. This type of hypnosis is often used to change behaviors and habits, improve sports performance, manage pain, reduce stress and anxiety, and treat conditions like phobias and neuroses. However, only about 20-30% of people respond well to this form of hypnosis.

Ericksonian Hypnosis

Named after Dr. Milton Erickson, this type of hypnosis is non-directive. Instead of giving commands, the therapist uses metaphors, stories, and indirect suggestions tailored to the individual's needs. This method is flexible and allows the client to feel independent and in control. Ericksonian hypnosis is particularly effective for people resistant to traditional methods and can help with anxiety, phobias, and changing negative habits. It's also easily integrated with other therapies like cognitive behavioral therapy.

Pharmacological Hypnosis

Pharmacological hypnosis involves using medications to achieve a hypnotic state. These drugs can help induce a deeper trance or control pain. This type of hypnosis is often used in medical settings, such as during surgeries or in treatments for addictions to alcohol, drugs, nicotine, or food.

Stage Hypnosis

Stage or pop hypnosis is used for entertainment. The hypnotist performs a pre-planned act to amuse the audience. It's about making people laugh, not achieving any therapeutic goals.

Self-Hypnosis

Self-hypnosis is a technique where a person hypnotizes themselves without external help. Using relaxation techniques and visualization, they enter a state of deep concentration similar to a hypnotic trance. In this state, they can use positive affirmations or visualize goals to bring about positive changes in thoughts, behaviors, and emotions. Self-hypnosis can reduce stress, boost confidence, overcome fears, and motivate personal growth. It requires practice and patience but can be a powerful tool for self-improvement.

Each type of hypnosis has its own benefits and challenges. With the right approach, hypnosis can be an effective way to achieve various personal and therapeutic goals.

When is Hypnosis Used?

Hypnosis is a powerful tool that can help with many different problems. Here are some of the most common ways it is used:

- Treating addictions: Helping people overcome addictions to substances like drugs or alcohol.
- Weight management: Assisting in weight loss and developing healthier eating habits.
- Reducing anxiety and stress: Lowering anxiety levels and helping people manage stress better.
- Overcoming phobias and fears: Addressing specific fears, such as fear of flying or public speaking.
- Improving sleep: Helping with sleep disorders like insomnia.
- Relieving pain: Managing chronic pain or pain from injuries.

- Boosting self-esteem: Increasing confidence and self-worth.
- Enhancing performance: Improving focus and performance in activities like sports or academics.
- Healing from trauma: Aiding in recovery from psychological trauma and emotional distress.

Hypnosis is used by various professionals, including hypnotherapists (who have special training and certification in hypnosis), coaches, psychiatrists, psychotherapists, and psychologists.

If you are interested in exploring new ways to solve problems or looking for personal and professional development, consider taking intensive psychology courses. These courses typically last from two weeks to a few months and can help you understand topics of interest, update your knowledge, or increase your skills.

Who Should Not Use Hypnosis?

While hypnosis can be helpful, it's not suitable for everyone. People with the following conditions should avoid hypnosis:

- Under the influence of alcohol or drugs.
- Suffering from severe mental disorders such as bipolar disorder or schizophrenia.
- Taking medications like antidepressants, sedatives, or antipsychotics.
- Having a history of heart attacks or strokes.
- Experiencing a concussion or high fever.
- Living with epilepsy or severe developmental delays.
- Being in early childhood.

Always consult with a specialist to avoid any unwanted effects.

How Does a Hypnotherapy Session Work?

A typical hypnosis session includes several steps to help you achieve a state of focused attention and relaxation:

1. Identifying the Issue: The session starts with discussing the problem. The hypnotherapist observes the person's speech and values to understand what is important to them and explains the purpose of the sessions.

2. Inducing Trance: The next step involves entering a trance state. The hypnotherapist might use techniques like the "Mobius House" to help the person become deeply relaxed and focused.

3. Deepening the Trance: The hypnotherapist helps the person go into a deeper trance using methods like counting or guided visualization, such as imagining walking down a staircase.

4. Therapeutic Intervention: In this phase, the therapist works with images and metaphors that can help improve the person's condition.

5. Post-Hypnotic Suggestion: This involves giving suggestions that will stay with the person after the session, helping them to maintain the benefits of the therapy.

6. Waking Up: The session ends with the therapist gently bringing the person out of the trance, often by counting or using

calming suggestions. Afterward, the person may feel refreshed and relaxed.

The specific steps and techniques can vary depending on the therapist's approach and the individual's needs. Hypnosis is a collaborative process, and the person's openness and willingness to participate are crucial for the session's success.

Pros and Cons of Hypnosis

Pros:

- Effective for changing habits: Hypnosis can help you overcome bad habits and unwanted behaviors.
- Access to the subconscious: It allows you to explore and resolve deep-seated issues.
- Personalized treatment: Hypnotherapy is tailored to each person's unique needs.
- Non-invasive: It's a treatment method that doesn't involve drugs and can be an alternative when medications aren't suitable.
- Combines well with other therapies: It can enhance the effectiveness of other treatment methods.

Cons:

- Varies in effectiveness: Hypnotherapy's success can depend on the individual.

- Limited scientific support: There is some skepticism due to limited scientific data backing its effectiveness.
- Requires trust: The success of sessions may rely on how much the client trusts the therapist.
- Misconceptions: Some people mistakenly view hypnotherapy as mere entertainment, which can deter them from trying it.
- Not for everyone: There are restrictions and contraindications that make hypnosis unsuitable for certain individuals.

How To Tell If Someone Is Hypnotized

Hypnosis affects people differently, so it's important to know how to recognize if someone is in a hypnotic state. Here are some signs that can indicate if someone is hypnotized:

Change in Pulse or Heart Rate

When someone is in hypnosis, they often become very relaxed, and their pulse rate tends to slow down, just like in any relaxed state. You can usually check their pulse rate at the side of their neck where the carotid artery is. However, if they're doing something active or thinking about something stressful, their pulse might go up.

Confused or Thoughtful Appearance

People in hypnosis might look confused, deep in thought, or have a blank expression.

This happens because they're not fully aware of their surroundings or not reacting as they usually would.

Less Response to External Stimuli
One way to tell if someone is in hypnosis is by noticing how they react to things around them. Usually, when someone is hypnotized, they are less bothered by external things like noises. For example, if there's a loud noise, someone not in hypnosis might jump, but a hypnotized person probably won't react much. This is because they are very focused and might be more engaged in their imagination, blocking out outside distractions. You can test this by making a noise and seeing if they react.

Glazed Eyes

If a person is hypnotized and you ask them to open their eyes, they might look like they just woke up. Their eyes might look glazed or slightly red, and they may seem like they are staring into space. This is similar to how someone looks when they wake up from a nap.

Hypnotic Phenomena

To see if someone is really in hypnosis, you can test for certain hypnotic responses. For example, you can check if they show signs of catalepsy (where they hold a position without moving), amnesia (forgetting things), analgesia (not feeling pain), hallucinations (seeing or hearing things that aren't there), or unconscious movements. Testing these responses helps you understand how deep the person is in hypnosis.

Recognizing these signs can help you determine if someone is in a hypnotic state and how deep they are in the trance.

Increased Focus

When someone is hypnotized, they show a heightened level of concentration. They listen closely to the hypnotist's words and suggestions, ignoring other thoughts and distractions around them. It's clear they are deeply involved in what the hypnotist is saying and using their imagination to follow instructions.

Eyes Watering (Lacrimation)

During hypnosis, a person's eyes might water even if they're not crying. This is called lacrimation and can happen without any emotional trigger. If you see this, it's a good idea to ask them, "How are you feeling right now?" If they mention feeling relaxed or calm, it's probably just a physical reaction to being in hypnosis. If they talk about emotions, then it might be related to something they are feeling during the session.

Muscular Relaxation

One of the most common signs of hypnosis is muscle relaxation. When people are deeply relaxed, their muscles become loose. This is why you might see people slumping over during stage hypnosis shows or in therapy sessions. A person might start sitting upright, but as they relax, their head and shoulders may droop forward. You might also notice their facial muscles relaxing, making them look younger and smoothing out wrinkles.

Random Muscle Spasms

Sometimes, a hypnotized person might have small or large muscle spasms, called myoclonic jerks. These are involuntary twitches that can happen in different parts of the body, like the muscles around the mouth or even an entire arm. This is similar to the sudden jerks people experience when they are falling asleep.

Rapid Eye Movement (REM) and Eye Fluttering

Rapid eye movement is a clear sign of hypnosis. It occurs when someone is visualizing something in their mind. This is similar to the rapid eye movement seen during sleep and dreaming. You might notice their eyes moving under their eyelids, as if they're looking around in an imaginary scene, or see their eyelids fluttering.

Skin Color Changes

When someone is in hypnosis, their skin color might change. They could become paler or their skin might flush. This change in skin color is a good indicator that they are in a hypnotic state. You can even suggest to them to feel warmer or cooler to see if their skin color responds accordingly.

Slowed Breathing

People in hypnosis often breathe more slowly. Since hypnosis promotes deep relaxation, their breathing rate can decrease significantly. While an awake adult usually breathes 12 to 16 times per minute, a hypnotized person might breathe as slowly as 3 to 6 times per minute.

These signs can help you tell if someone is in hypnosis. Increased focus, muscle relaxation, slower breathing, and other changes are good indicators that someone is deeply relaxed and hypnotized. Not all signs will be present in everyone, but noticing even a few can show that a person is in a hypnotic state.

Slowed Physical Responses

When someone is deeply hypnotized, they usually move more slowly. If you ask a person in hypnosis to lift a hand, move a finger, or nod in response to a question, they might take longer than usual to do so. This slow reaction can indicate they are in a hypnotic state.

You might also notice that a hypnotized person takes longer to speak. This happens often in hypnotherapy sessions because the topics discussed require more time for subconscious processing, unlike stage hypnosis, which is designed for quick responses.

Slower Blink Rate and Longer Blinks

If you have someone open their eyes while they are still in hypnosis, you might notice their blink rate has slowed down and each blink lasts longer. This is another good sign that they are hypnotized.

Stillness

Catalepsy, or a state of stillness, can occur during hypnosis. Some people might remain completely still and immobile without moving or shifting to get comfortable, unlike when they are awake and resting. This is a natural response in hypnosis and can be more noticeable as the session goes on, unless the person is actively moving during the hypnosis.

Change in Swallowing Rate

In hypnosis, some people might notice a change in how often they swallow. Some produce more saliva and swallow more frequently, while others might experience a dry mouth and swallow less often. To observe this, you need to know their usual swallowing rate before they go into hypnosis so you can compare it to their swallowing rate during hypnosis.

Tendency to Agree and Follow Suggestions

A good way to tell if someone is hypnotized is to see if they are agreeing with and following the hypnotist's suggestions. Hypnotized people are more likely to go along with what is suggested to them. If someone isn't following the suggestions or seems distracted, they might not be fully hypnotized. For some purposes, light hypnosis might be enough, but for others, deeper hypnosis might be required. Testing how suggestible someone is can be a useful way to gauge their level of hypnosis.

Summary

Watching for slowed movements, slower blinking, stillness, changes in swallowing, and a tendency to agree with suggestions can help you tell if someone is hypnotized. Each person may show these signs differently, but these cues can help you determine if someone is in a hypnotic state.

Chapter 2

The Power of Self-Hypnosis

Self-hypnosis is a fascinating concept that has shown impressive results in various situations. Medical history even records instances where people died because of strong suggestions or self-hypnosis. For example, an English physiologist named Cannon observed a case where healthy young tribe members in Africa died after breaking a taboo. The shaman declared a death sentence for violating the taboo, and even before any physical punishment was carried out, the individuals died because their hearts simply stopped. This phenomenon is sometimes referred to as "shamanic death."

Can We Control Our Own Bodies?

A key question that arises is whether we can consciously influence our own body and nervous system using self-suggestion. Can we manage our fears, reduce anxiety and stress, control heart and blood vessel functions, regulate pain, change our body temperature, and even improve our memory and attention? In other words, can we achieve conscious control over our bodily processes that we typically consider beyond our control? Is it possible to improve our health and well-being through self-hypnosis?

The answer, according to some systems like yoga and modern science, is a firm "yes." By learning techniques of psychophysiological self-regulation and active self-hypnosis, we can indeed influence our health.

The Emile Coue Method

In the 1920s, the self-hypnosis method developed by French psychiatrist Emile Coue became very popular. Coue believed that the human imagination was a major factor in illness, and therefore he proposed treating people through self-hypnosis. He suggested that patients sit in a comfortable position and repeatedly say positive affirmations, either mentally or in a whisper, 30 times in a row, several times a day.

One of the most famous affirmations Coue recommended was, "Every day, in every way, I am getting better and better." Other examples include, "I feel stronger every day," or "My vision (or hearing, or other functions) is improving," and "I am completely healthy."

The Impact of Self-Hypnosis

Self-hypnosis can have a significant impact on various bodily functions, especially for people with vivid imaginations. There are many documented cases of false pregnancies, where a person exhibits all the external signs of pregnancy purely due to the power of belief. Similarly, self-hypnosis can affect the regulation of blood vessels and other body functions.

How Self-Hypnosis Works

To understand how suggestion and self-suggestion work, we need to recognize that our unconscious mind controls all our bodily functions. If we can convince our unconscious mind that our body should heal itself, it will start the process of recovery. The body will either quickly or gradually return to its normal state, depending on the situation.

This concept helps explain how self-hypnosis can stop bleeding, heal burns, reduce swelling, and treat other conditions like paralysis, ulcers, and wounds. For example, stopping bleeding through self-hypnosis might seem extraordinary, but it's actually straightforward. The unconscious mind sends signals to the veins and arteries to constrict and stop the bleeding, similar to how adrenaline works as a hemostatic agent.

Reducing swelling works in much the same way. When the unconscious mind accepts the idea that the swelling should decrease, it signals the brain to constrict the blood vessels supplying the swollen area.

Self-Hypnosis in Medical Treatments
Self-hypnosis has been known to achieve remarkable results, even in cases like cancer treatment. In medicine, the placebo effect—where patients get better after taking a sugar pill—illustrates the power of self-hypnosis and belief.

However, some biologists argue that humans have lost the ability to directly influence their bodies with thought due to evolutionary changes. They believe that self-hypnosis might not be as effective as some people claim.

Regardless of differing opinions, the potential of self-hypnosis as a tool for personal health and well-being remains an intriguing and powerful area of exploration.

How to Hypnotize

Hypnotizing someone involves a series of steps to guide them into a relaxed state of focused attention. Here are five simple steps to help you learn how to hypnotize someone:

Step 1: Building Rapport

Start by building rapport with the person you're hypnotizing. This involves creating a comfortable atmosphere and understanding their goals or issues they want to address. Ask questions to gain insights into their language and concerns. Building rapport sets the stage for a successful hypnosis session.

Step 2: Hypnotic Induction and Deepening

Begin the induction process by gaining the person's consent to engage in hypnosis.

Using techniques like Rapid Eye Movement (R.E.M), guide them into a trance state characterized by increased relaxation and focus. Deepen the trance gradually using calming phrases and a soothing voice. Pay attention to subtle signs of relaxation.

Step 3: Recognizing Signs of Hypnosis

During hypnosis, look for signs like tearing of the eyes, rapid eye movement under the eyelids, changes in skin color, altered breathing rhythm, or slight body movements. These signs indicate that the person is in a trance state. Remember, not everyone exhibits the same signs, so be observant.

Step 4: Envisioning the Future

After guiding the person through the main part of the session, it's time to focus on their future desired state. Encourage them to imagine achieving their goals or reaching their desired outcome. This involves visualizing themselves in a few months, having already made the changes they desire.

Helping someone envision their future success can be done in various ways, such as picturing themselves in a winner's circle or visualizing their ideal size and shape. By visualizing success, the subconscious mind can be directed towards achieving the desired outcome.

Step 5: Reinforcing Suggestions

Finally, it's essential to reinforce the positive suggestions made during the session. Repeat affirmations like "Your mind is focused and clear" or affirm that the suggestions are deeply embedded in the subconscious mind and will grow stronger over time.

Ending the Session

When concluding the hypnosis session, ensure a gradual return to full consciousness. Avoid abruptly pulling the person out of the hypnotic state. Slowly make them aware of their surroundings using verbal cues. For example, you can say, "I will count to five, and when I reach five, you will be fully awake again."

If possible, discuss the session with the person afterward to gather feedback. Ask about their experience during hypnosis, including any feelings of being pulled back to wakefulness. This feedback can help improve future sessions and provide a better experience for the individual.

Chapter 3

Understanding Hypnotherapy

Hypnotherapy, when used correctly by a specialist, can be a powerful tool for addressing various neurotic disorders. Historically, it's one of the earliest methods used in psychiatry, with its roots tracing back to the work of German doctor Franz Anton Mesmer (1734-1815). Initially, it was based on the theory of influencing bodily fluids through classical hypnosis. Later, in the 1920s, Milton Erickson (1900-1985), another prominent figure, introduced Ericksonian hypnosis, which revolutionized hypnotherapy by emphasizing innovative suggestion techniques.

What is Hypnotherapy?

Hypnotherapy essentially refers to using hypnosis as a form of treatment. There are two main approaches: classical hypnosis and Ericksonian hypnosis. The core of hypnotherapy involves inducing a person into a unique state of consciousness known as trance. Trance is akin to a blend of wakefulness and sleep, where the body rests while the mind remains alert, immersed in dreamlike imagery. In this state, individuals are highly receptive to the therapist's words, experiencing heightened suggestibility. This power of suggestion within trance facilitates therapeutic effects, making hypnotherapy an effective intervention for various conditions.

The Difference Between Classical and Ericksonian Hypnosis

Hypnosis techniques can vary widely, but two primary methods are classical and Ericksonian hypnosis. Understanding their differences can help in choosing the most suitable approach for therapy.

Classical Hypnosis

Classical hypnosis typically involves a therapist guiding the patient into a trance state using direct commands, often culminating in the instruction to "Sleep!" This method emphasizes authority and aims to induce a rapid state of altered consciousness. Suggestion formulas used in classical hypnosis are straightforward and direct, focusing on commands like "Hands relax and become heavier" or "Plunge into a pleasant, comfortable relaxing state."

Ericksonian Hypnosis

In contrast, Ericksonian hypnosis employs a smoother, gentler approach to induction. Therapists take a collaborative stance, guiding patients into trance more subtly. Suggestions in Ericksonian hypnosis are mostly indirect, utilizing open suggestions, implications, and other techniques to engage the patient's imagination. For instance, phrases like "Your deep mind can find all the necessary resources" or "It's similar to that feeling when your mind is awake and your body is asleep" are common.

Utilization Principle

Another significant difference lies in the principle of utilization. Ericksonian hypnotherapy relies on harnessing the patient's own resources, such as memories or latent abilities, to facilitate healing. In contrast, classical hypnosis often focuses more on prescribing therapeutic suggestions directly.

In essence, the distinction between classical and Ericksonian hypnotherapy lies in their approach to patient cooperation. Ericksonian hypnosis emphasizes collaboration and resource utilization, while classical hypnosis leans towards direct suggestion and authority.

Additional Note

It's worth noting the concept of everyday trance, which many people experience without realizing it. This mild trance state occurs during activities like daydreaming or getting lost in thought, akin to focusing on passing scenery during a commute. Understanding these natural trance states can demystify hypnosis, highlighting its innate familiarity rather than the dramatic portrayals often seen in media.

Degrees of Hypnotic Trance

Before delving into hypnotherapy sessions, it's essential to grasp the varying levels of trance, categorized into three stages:

1. Light Trance: Characterized by feelings of relaxation and internal focus, individuals remain fully aware and can easily open their eyes if needed.

2. Medium Trance: In this state, bodily sensations intensify, including feelings of heaviness or lightness, sometimes accompanied by sensations of flying or forgetfulness.

3. Deep Trance: Also known as somnambulistic trance, this level involves profound immersion into the subconscious, often resulting in complete amnesia for the session upon awakening. Deep trance can facilitate regression therapy or profound insights but may require careful guidance for safe navigation.

Understanding these levels of trance can help therapists tailor hypnotherapy sessions to suit individual needs effectively.

How a Hypnotherapy Session Works

Hypnotherapy sessions involve several stages to guide individuals into a state of trance and utilize therapeutic interventions effectively. Here's a breakdown of the seven stages typically involved:

1. Induction and Formation of Trance Signs

The session begins with induction, a technique to induce trance. This can involve visual or auditory methods, such as focusing on an object or counting. The goal is to separate from the external environment and distractions.

2. Deepening Trance

Deepening the trance enhances the effectiveness of therapy by allowing for more vivid perception of unconscious processes. This can be achieved through counting, imagery, or figurative techniques, guiding the individual into a deeper state of relaxation.

3. Therapeutic Intervention

The main part of the session involves therapeutic intervention, where the therapist works with suggested images or metaphors related to the individual's issues. Techniques like dispersion, introduced by Milton Erickson, use indirect metaphors to lay down subconscious meanings for further work.

4. Therapeutic Suggestion

Therapeutic suggestion follows the intervention, aiming to maintain the effects achieved. These suggestions can be direct or indirect, focusing on stabilizing the individual's condition and reinforcing positive changes.

5. Post-hypnotic Suggestion

Post-hypnotic suggestion adds to the therapeutic suggestions by addressing future behaviors. These suggestions often outline new behavioral strategies to implement after the session, such as coping mechanisms for anxiety.

6. Creating Amnesia

In some cases, amnesia is induced before exiting the trance to prevent the individual from criticizing or undermining the effectiveness of the suggestions. This helps consolidate the therapeutic results deep within the unconscious mind.

7. Breaking Out of Trance

Finally, the session concludes with a smooth transition out of the trance state. This can be signaled by the individual's readiness or through a countdown. It's crucial to ensure a gentle exit to avoid any unpleasant sensations.

Understanding these stages can demystify hypnotherapy sessions and highlight their structured approach to facilitating positive changes in individuals' lives.

Hypnosis Indications

Hypnotherapy offers effective solutions for various conditions, particularly addiction and psychosomatic disorders.

Addiction Management

Hypnosis can aid in managing addictions like alcohol, smoking, or eating disorders. Through tailored programs, it helps reduce cravings and develops new behaviors to overcome addictive patterns.

Psychosomatic Disorders

Psychosomatic disorders involve bodily sensations without an organic basis, such as unexplained changes in blood pressure, headaches, or motor issues despite physical health. Hypnotherapy can address these symptoms by identifying their underlying causes and providing targeted intervention.

Identifying Root Causes

Hypnosis serves as a potent method to pinpoint internal issues' origins and resolve them. By inducing a trance state, it brings awareness to underlying problems, facilitating effective therapy.

Conclusion

When administered by a skilled professional, hypnotherapy proves to be a valuable tool in treating various neurotic disorders. Its ability to uncover root causes and provide targeted solutions makes it a powerful therapeutic approach.

Chapter 4

Hypnotic Trance

Misconceptions about Trance

Many people misunderstand hypnotic trance, fearing it as a state where someone else controls their actions against their will. This misconception prevents them from recognizing its empowering potential.

Understanding Trance

Trance isn't about losing control; it's a state of mind with vast possibilities for self-exploration and problem-solving. It enhances performance in tasks and enriches daily experiences.

Accessing Trance

Trance is a natural human ability, accessible to almost everyone. Recognizing that it's within your control raises the question: why not explore its benefits?

Trance in History and Culture

Trance has been part of human consciousness for ages. It's a biological mechanism evolved for survival, adaptable to individual and societal needs. Importantly, all hypnosis is self-hypnosis.

Biological and Social Aspects

Trance is influenced by both biology and society. Dissociation and absorption are inherent to individuals, while suggestibility is shaped by social and cultural factors.

Conclusion

Trance, a blend of biological and social elements, offers immense potential for personal growth. Understanding its nature empowers individuals to harness its benefits and enrich their lives.

Exploring Dissociation, Absorption, and Suggestibility

Dissociation: Tuning Out
Dissociation is when you disconnect from the world around you, like daydreaming or zoning out. It's a way our minds take a break from reality, often during stressful times. Some can do this easily, while others find it hard.

Absorption: Getting Lost
Absorption is diving deep into an activity, like reading or watching a movie, so much that you lose track of time and the world around you. It's a skill that varies from person to person.

Suggestibility: Going with the Flow

Suggestibility is about being open to others' ideas and fitting into social norms. It's not about being gullible but adapting to what's expected in a group.

The Power of Trance

Trance, a mix of dissociation and absorption, is a common human experience. We all slip into it now and then, especially during daydreaming. Learning to use trance deliberately can help solve problems and improve various aspects of life.

Embracing Trance

Harnessing the power of trance is a skill anyone can learn. By understanding how our minds work in dissociation and absorption, we can tap into this natural ability to make positive changes and grow.

Exploring Different Depths of Hypnosis

Everyone experiences hypnosis differently. Some people can reach deep states of hypnosis, while others stay in a lighter state. But here's the thing: whether it's deep or light, you can still benefit from it if you're open to relaxing and listening.

The Depth of Trance States:

1. Light Trance: Almost everyone can achieve this level, which is like deep relaxation with focused attention. Some say it's not very useful, but with well-crafted suggestions, it can help you achieve a lot. It's not just about being hypnotized; it's about the therapy within the hypnotic state that brings results.

2. Apparent Somnambulism: This state looks like true somnambulism from the outside, but it's not the same. While true somnambulism can induce deep anesthesia for surgeries, apparent somnambulism isn't deep enough for that. Even small things like a pin prick might cause a reaction, but the person is still hypnotized, just not as deeply as in light trance.

3. True Somnambulism

True somnambulism is a state where both the mind and body are completely relaxed. Some therapists believe it's essential for effective suggestion because it creates a state of 'blankness' where the mind is so relaxed that it can't resist suggestions. In this state, it's possible to create anesthesia strong enough for surgeries, like open-heart surgery. While not everyone can reach this depth, it's remarkable what can be achieved with proper use of hypnosis.

4. Coma State (or Esdaile State)

The coma state, also known as the Esdaile state, is deeper than somnambulism. It's characterized by a feeling of bliss and euphoria, with little concern about surroundings. Major surgeries can be performed in this state, and the individual only experiences what they wish to feel. While it's assumed that suggestions might be more effective here, there's little evidence to support this. Also, this ultra-deep level isn't necessary for effective self-hypnosis.

How Deep Can You Go?

The depth of your hypnosis experience varies from person to person. You don't need to reach the level required for surgeries in our self-hypnosis recordings. A light trance state, which most people can achieve, is perfectly suitable. Remember, while hypnosis plays a role, it's the therapy within the hypnotic state that brings about change.